MY CARDIO HEALTH

Guidelines to a healthy heart

Dr. FREDERICK BOLY

Copyright

No part of this book should be copied, reproduced without the author's permission @2023 Cardiovascular Chronicles by Dr. Frederick Boly

TABLE OF CONTENT

Introduction

The Importance of Cardiovascular Health
Cardiovascular health is crucial since it has a direct impact on a person's general wellbeing. The lifeline of the human body is the cardiovascular system, which includes the heart and blood vessels and is essential in delivering oxygen and nutrition to all body cells. It is essential to comprehend its significance.

First and foremost, a strong cardiovascular system ensures that the brain, muscles, and organs receive adequate oxygenation. This oxygen is essential for the synthesis of energy, which enables us to go about our daily lives with vigor. Along with supporting physical health, it also aids in cognitive function, memory, and alertness.

The key to longevity is also maintaining cardiovascular health. The major causes of death worldwide are cardiac disorders such coronary artery disease and heart attacks. Taking a heart-healthy lifestyle

What Is a Healthy Heart?

The cornerstone of general health is the heart, the body's main pump that continuously circulates blood throughout the entire system to sustain life. The size of a clenched fist, this extraordinary organ has four chambers: two atria and two ventricles, all of which work in perfect harmony.

Efficiency is an essential part of a healthy heart. It absorbs blood that has lost oxygen for reoxygenation in the lungs while also pumping blood that is nutrient- and oxygen-rich to vital organs, tissues, and cells. Through this process, the body's cells receive the vital nutrients they need to function at their best.

Clear, unobstructed blood vessels are also necessary for a healthy heart. The health of arteries, veins, and capillaries depends on their ability to

Goals of This Book

1. Comprehensive Education: Give readers a thorough understanding of the cardiovascular system's structure, operation, and relationship to general health.

2. Disease Prevention: Provide readers with useful tips and methods to lower their risk of cardiovascular illnesses by making lifestyle adjustments such dietary, physical activity, and stress reduction.

3. Early Detection: Inform readers about the value of routine checkups, screenings, and self-evaluation. You should also provide advice on when to seek medical assistance.

4. Treatment Options: Explore different treatment techniques, from drugs to surgeries, in a straightforward and transparent manner to help readers make judgments.

5: Practical Advice: To offer readers practical advice on how to enhance their cardiovascular health, including dietary adjustments, exercise regimens, and stress reduction approaches.

6: Risk Assessment: To assist readers in identifying and understanding their own personal cardiovascular risk factors.

7: Holistic Approach: To highlight the value of a holistic approach to health, which includes mental and emotional well-being, in preserving a healthy heart.

8: Lifetime Learning: To inspire a commitment to lifetime learning by encouraging readers to keep up with the most recent advancements in cardiovascular health and research.

9: Inspirational Stories: To share true accounts of people who have successfully dealt with or overcame cardiovascular issues in order to inspire and offer hope.

Chapter 1

Understanding the Cardiovascular System

The cardiovascular framework, frequently alluded to as the circulatory framework, is a perplexing organization of organs, vessels, and cells that assumes an essential part in supporting life. Its essential capability is to ship blood, which conveys oxygen, supplements, chemicals, and byproducts, all through the body. Understanding this framework is fundamental for valuing its importance in keeping up with generally speaking wellbeing.

At the center of the cardiovascular framework is the heart, a strong organ about the size of a clench hand, which goes about as a strong siphon. It comprises of four chambers: two atria and two ventricles. The atria get blood from different pieces of the body, while the ventricles siphon it out. This organized siphoning activity creates the fundamental power to move blood through the supply routes, which divert oxygen-rich blood from the heart to the body's tissues and organs.

On the other hand, veins get oxygen-drained blood from the body once again to the heart. The predominant vena cava gathers blood from the chest area, while the mediocre vena cava assembles it from the lower body. Blood from both is then siphoned into the right chamber and accordingly into the right ventricle prior to being shipped off the lungs for oxygenation.

The left half of the heart gets oxygenated blood from the lungs and siphons it into the aorta, the biggest corridor in the body. This aorta branches into more modest corridors, which further gap into little vessels. These vessels take into account the trading of oxygen and supplements with the body's cells, all the while eliminating side-effects like carbon dioxide.

Keeping a sound cardiovascular framework is central to in general prosperity. Factors like a fair eating routine, standard activity, and keeping away from tobacco and extreme liquor utilization can assist with forestalling cardiovascular infections like hypertension, atherosclerosis, and coronary episodes. Ordinary check-ups with medical services experts can support early recognition and the board of possible issues. Understanding the cardiovascular framework's many-sided operations engages people to go with informed way of life decisions, encouraging a more drawn out, better life.

Anatomy of the Heart

The heart, an imperative organ in the circulatory framework, is a solid, four-chambered structure situated in the chest. It assumes a focal part in siphoning blood all through the body.

The heart comprises of two primary parts: the right and left sides, each separated into two chambers. The right chamber gets deoxygenated blood from the body through the unrivaled and second rate vena cava, while the right ventricle siphons this blood to the lungs for oxygenation.

On the left side, the left chamber gets oxygen-rich blood from the lungs through the pneumonic veins. The left ventricle then powerfully discharges this oxygenated blood into the aorta, which conveys it to the whole body.

Valves inside the heart, like the tricuspid and bicuspid (mitral) valves, forestall discharge of blood between chambers. The heart's cadenced withdrawals are directed by an electrical framework, including the sinoatrial (SA) hub and atrioventricular (AV) hub.

Coronary courses supply the heart muscle with oxygen and supplements, guaranteeing its appropriate capability. Any disturbance in this blood supply can prompt coronary illness.

In outline, the heart's four chambers, valves, electrical framework, and coronary veins work amicably to course oxygenated blood to the body and deoxygenated blood to the lungs, supporting in general physical processes.

Function of the Heart

The heart, often described as a muscular pump, is the central component of the circulatory system, and its primary function is to circulate blood throughout the body. This vital organ ensures that oxygen and nutrients reach every cell while removing waste products.

The heart has four chambers: two atria (upper chambers) and two ventricles (lower chambers). Its function can be summarized in a series of steps:

1. Blood Collection: Deoxygenated blood, which has delivered its oxygen to the body's cells, returns to the right atrium from the body via two major veins: the superior and inferior vena cava.

2. Pumping to the Lungs: The right atrium contracts, pushing blood into the right ventricle. When the right ventricle contracts, it pumps this deoxygenated blood through the pulmonary valve into the pulmonary artery, leading to the lungs. In the lungs, blood picks up oxygen and releases carbon dioxide.

3. Oxygenated Blood Return: Oxygen-rich blood returns to the left atrium through the pulmonary veins. The left atrium contracts, pushing this blood into the left ventricle.

4. Systemic Circulation: The left ventricle, being the strongest chamber, pumps oxygenated blood through the aortic valve into the aorta—the body's largest artery. From there, the aorta branches out, delivering oxygen and nutrients to every organ and tissue.

5. Continuous Cycle: This oxygenated blood travels through smaller arteries and arterioles, eventually reaching tiny capillaries where oxygen and nutrients are exchanged for waste products. Deoxygenated blood, now loaded with waste, flows into veins and returns to the heart, starting the cycle again.

The heart's rhythm is controlled by electrical signals generated by the sinoatrial (SA) node, the heart's natural pacemaker. The atrioventricular (AV) node regulates the timing of contractions between the atria and ventricles.

In essence, the heart's function is to ensure the continuous flow of blood, supplying oxygen and nutrients to sustain the body's functions while simultaneously removing waste and carbon dioxide, thereby supporting overall health and vitality.

Blood Vessels and Circulation

Blood vessels are like highways that transport blood throughout your body. There are three main types:

1. Arteries: These resemble the thruways leaving a city, conveying oxygen-rich blood from the heart to all aspects of your body. The biggest course is the aorta, which branches into more modest conduits.

2. Veins: Veins resemble the streets taking traffic back to the city. They convey deoxygenated blood, brimming with waste and carbon dioxide, from your body's tissues back to the heart. The biggest vein, the predominant and mediocre vena cava, returns blood to the heart.

3. Capillaries: Vessels are little, limited streets that associate corridors to veins, similar to little roads in an area. They're where the genuine activity occurs. Supplements, oxygen, and waste are traded among blood and cells through their slim walls.

Together, these veins make up your circulatory framework, guaranteeing a consistent progression of blood to support your body and eliminate squander. A tremendous organization keeps you perfectly healthy.

Chapter 2

Coronary illness is a main source of disease and demise around the world, and understanding its gamble factors is significant for counteraction and the executives. A few variables add to an expanded gamble of coronary illness, some of which can be controlled or changed, while others are past our impact. Here are key gamble factors:

1. Hypertension :Raised pulse powers the heart to work harder, prompting likely harm to veins and the actual heart. Uncontrolled hypertension is a huge gamble factor for coronary illness.

2. High Cholesterol: Elevated degrees of LDL cholesterol (frequently called "awful" cholesterol) can prompt plaque development in veins, limiting them and expanding the gamble of coronary course illness.

3. Smoking: Tobacco smoke contains unsafe synthetics that harm veins and increment the gamble of atherosclerosis (solidifying of the courses), making smoking a significant supporter of coronary illness.

4. Diabetes: Uncontrolled diabetes can harm veins and nerves, expanding the gamble of coronary illness. Individuals with diabetes have a higher possibility encountering coronary episodes and strokes.

5. Obesity: Overabundance body weight, especially around the midsection, is related with worse hypertension, cholesterol levels, and an expanded gamble of coronary illness.

6. Actual Inactivity: A stationary way of life adds to weight and raises the gamble of coronary illness. Ordinary active work keeps a sound weight and works on cardiovascular wellbeing.

7. Poor Diet: Consuming an eating routine high in immersed and trans fats, sodium (salt), and refined sugars can prompt heftiness, hypertension, and elevated cholesterol, expanding coronary illness risk.

8. Family History: A family background of coronary illness, particularly in the event that it happened quite early on, can raise your gamble. Hereditary qualities can assume a part in coronary illness powerlessness.

9. Age: As individuals age, the gamble of coronary illness increments. Men more than 45 and ladies north of 55 are at higher gamble.

10. Gender: Men by and large have a higher gamble of coronary illness contrasted with premenopausal ladies. Notwithstanding, the gamble turns out to be more comparable after menopause.

11. Stress: Ongoing pressure can add to coronary illness risk by prompting undesirable adapting ways of behaving like indulging, smoking, or inordinate drinking.

12. Liquor Consumption: Unnecessary liquor admission can raise pulse, add to stoutness, and lead to heart muscle harm. Balance is vital.

Understanding these gamble factors engages people to make way of life changes and look for clinical direction to decrease their gamble of coronary illness. Ordinary check-ups, a heart-solid eating regimen, work out, and not smoking are significant stages toward a better heart and a more drawn out, really satisfying life.

Genetics and Family History

Genetics assumes a huge part in the gamble of cardiovascular sicknesses (CVDs). On the off chance that you have a family background of specific cardiovascular sicknesses, your hereditary inclination could expand your powerlessness to these circumstances. Here are a few instances of cardiovascular sicknesses with hereditary connections and normal family ancestry situations:

1. Coronary Supply route Sickness (CAD): Computer aided design happens when the veins providing the heart become limited or hindered. If your folks or direct relations (particularly early in life) have had respiratory failures, angina, or required heart strategies like angioplasty or sidestep a medical procedure, you might have a hereditary inclination to computer aided design.

2. Hypertension (High Blood Pressure): A family background of hypertension can essentially expand your gamble. In the event that your folks or kin have hypertension, you might be hereditarily inclined toward foster it also.

3. Stroke: Family background of stroke can be connected to an expanded gamble. Assuming your direct relations have experienced ischemic strokes (brought about by hindered corridors in the mind) or hemorrhagic strokes (brought about by draining in the cerebrum), your hereditary gamble might be higher.

4. Familial Hypercholesterolemia (FH): FH is an acquired condition portrayed by exceptionally elevated degrees of LDL cholesterol. On the off chance that a parent or grandparent had FH, you might acquire this hereditary inclination, which can prompt beginning stage coronary illness.

5. Arrhythmias: Some heart cadence issues, as atrial fibrillation or long QT disorder, can run in families because of hereditary changes. In the event that there's a background marked by these circumstances in your family, you might have an expanded gamble.

6. Cardiomyopathies: Hereditary changes can prompt circumstances like hypertrophic cardiomyopathy or expanded cardiomyopathy. Assuming a relative has been determined to have these circumstances, there might be a hereditary part that expands your gamble.

7. Fringe Corridor Illness (PAD): On the off chance that relatives have encountered Cushion, a condition where courses in the legs become restricted, it could recommend a hereditary inclination to vascular illnesses.

It's critical to take note of that having a family background of these circumstances doesn't ensure that you'll foster them, yet it demonstrates a higher gamble. Understanding your family ancestry permits you and your medical services supplier to come to informed conclusions about preventive measures, for example, way of life changes and early screening, to relieve your cardiovascular illness risk. Hereditary testing may likewise be viewed as now and again to recognize explicit hereditary changes related with these circumstances

Lifestyle Choices

Life style choices assume a critical part in deciding a singular's gamble of creating cardiovascular illnesses (CVDs). These decisions can significantly affect heart wellbeing, either improving or diminishing the probability of conditions like coronary corridor sickness, cardiovascular failures, and stroke. Here is a broad clarification of how certain way of life decisions can raise the gamble of CVDs:

1. Dietary Habits: An eating routine high in immersed and trans fats, cholesterol, and sodium can add to the improvement of CVDs. These components can prompt the development of plaque in the conduits, causing atherosclerosis and expanding the gamble of coronary illness. On the other hand, an eating routine wealthy in natural products, vegetables, entire grains, and incline proteins can diminish this gamble.

2. Actual Inactivity: Inactive ways of life are a critical gamble factor for CVDs. Standard actual work keeps a solid weight, control circulatory strain, further develop cholesterol levels, and improve generally cardiovascular wellness. Inertia, then again, can prompt weight and a higher gamble of coronary illness.

3. Smoking and Tobacco Use: Smoking is one of the most unfavorable way of life decisions for heart wellbeing. The synthetics in tobacco smoke harm veins, lessen oxygen conveyance to tissues, and raise pulse. Smokers are at a lot higher gamble of cardiovascular failures and strokes.

4. Extreme Liquor Consumption: Savoring liquor abundance can prompt hypertension, sporadic heart rhythms, cardiomyopathy, and even cardiovascular breakdown. While moderate liquor

utilization might have a few cardiovascular advantages, over the top drinking presents serious dangers.

5. Stoutness and Abundance Body Weight: Being overweight or large is firmly connected to CVDs. Abundance muscle to fat ratio can prompt hypertension, elevated cholesterol levels, and insulin obstruction, all of which add to coronary illness.

6. Stress Management: Ongoing pressure can prompt undesirable strategies for dealing with especially difficult times like indulging, smoking, or inordinate drinking, which increment the gamble of coronary illness. Stress chemicals can likewise affect the heart and veins.

7. Inadequately Oversaw Diabetes: Individuals with uncontrolled diabetes are at a higher gamble of CVDs. Raised glucose levels can harm veins and nerves, improving the probability of respiratory failures, strokes, and other cardiovascular complexities.

8. Rest Deprivation: Inadequate or low quality rest has been related with a higher gamble of coronary illness. Rest is fundamental for by and large wellbeing, including heart wellbeing, as it permits the body to fix and recover.

9. High Pressure Levels: Ongoing pressure can add to undesirable ways of behaving, for example, gorging or smoking, which are inconvenient to heart wellbeing. Furthermore, stress chemicals like cortisol can straightforwardly influence the heart and veins.

10. Medication and Substance Abuse: Illegal medication use, like cocaine or amphetamines, can cause respiratory failures, arrhythmias, and other cardiovascular issues. Substance misuse

can likewise prompt a scope of medical problems that by implication increment CVD risk.

All in all, way of life decisions altogether influence the gamble of cardiovascular sicknesses. Embracing a heart-sound way of life, including a decent eating routine, ordinary active work, evasion of tobacco and extreme liquor, stress the executives, and keeping a solid weight, can considerably decrease the gamble of creating CVDs. It's crucial for pursue informed decisions to safeguard your heart and generally prosperity. Normal check-ups with medical care suppliers can likewise help survey and deal with these dangers successfully.

Health Conditions

A few medical issue are related with an expanded gamble of cardiovascular infection (CVD). These circumstances can add to the improvement of heart-related issues, including coronary course infection, cardiovascular failures, and strokes. Here are some normal ailments that are critical gamble factors for CVD:

1. Hypertension (High Blood Pressure): Raised pulse overwhelms the heart and veins, expanding the gamble of atherosclerosis (limiting of courses), coronary episodes, and stroke.

2. Elevated Cholesterol (Dyslipidemia): Elevated degrees of LDL cholesterol (frequently alluded to as "awful" cholesterol) can prompt the development of plaque in the supply routes, raising the gamble of coronary vein illness and respiratory failures.

3. Diabetes: Individuals with diabetes are at a higher gamble of CVD on the grounds that high glucose levels can harm veins and nerves. Cardiovascular confusions, including coronary failures and strokes, are more normal in people with diabetes.

4. Obesity: Overabundance body weight, especially when it's concentrated around the midsection, is a critical gamble factor for CVD. Heftiness is connected to hypertension, elevated cholesterol levels, and insulin obstruction, all of which add to coronary illness.

5. Metabolic Syndrome: Metabolic disorder is a group of conditions that increment CVD risk. It incorporates corpulence, hypertension, raised glucose levels, and strange lipid profiles.

6. Persistent Kidney Illness (CKD): Kidney sickness can prompt an aggregation of byproducts and liquids in the body, adding to hypertension and an expanded gamble of coronary illness.

7. Fringe Course Sickness (PAD): Cushion happens when veins in the legs become restricted, diminishing blood stream. It is related with an expanded gamble of coronary illness and stroke.

8. Immune system Diseases: Conditions like rheumatoid joint pain and fundamental lupus erythematosus are related with irritation, which can influence veins and increment the gamble of CVD.

9. Rest Apnea: Rest apnea, a condition portrayed by breaks in breathing during rest, is connected to hypertension and a raised gamble of coronary illness.

10. Fiery Conditions: Persistent incendiary circumstances, like psoriasis, can add to irritation all through the body, possibly influencing veins and expanding CVD risk.

11. Family History: A family background of cardiovascular infections, particularly in the event that direct relations had coronary failures or strokes quite early on, can show a hereditary inclination that raises your gamble.

12. Emotional well-being Disorders: Conditions like melancholy, nervousness, and persistent pressure can prompt unfortunate ways of behaving (e.g., indulging, smoking) and may straightforwardly affect the cardiovascular framework.

13. Thrombophilias: Hereditary or procured conditions that increment the propensity to shape blood clumps can raise the gamble of cardiovascular failures and strokes.

It's fundamental to perceive these ailments and oversee them actually through clinical consideration, way of life changes, and, now and again, prescription. Tending to these gamble variables can altogether diminish the probability of creating cardiovascular illnesses and further develop by and large heart wellbeing. Customary check-ups with a medical services supplier are indispensable for observing and dealing with these circumstances.

Age and Gender

Age and gender are two critical risk factors that significantly influence an individual's susceptibility to heart disease, also known as cardiovascular disease (CVD). Understanding how these factors interplay with heart health is essential for effective prevention and management.

Age as a Risk Factor

Advancing age is a primary and non-modifiable risk factor for heart disease. The aging process itself brings about significant changes in the cardiovascular system, making it more vulnerable to heart-related conditions. These age-related changes include:

1. Arterial Stiffness: As people age, their arteries become less flexible and more rigid, a condition known as arteriosclerosis. This can lead to increased blood pressure, a significant risk factor for heart disease.

2. Atherosclerosis: Over time, plaque—a buildup of cholesterol, fat, and other substances—accumulates in the arteries, narrowing them and reducing blood flow. This age-related phenomenon is a major contributor to coronary artery disease.

3. Reduced Heart Function: The heart may undergo structural and functional changes with age, making it less efficient at pumping blood. This can contribute to heart failure and other cardiac issues.

4. Risk Accumulation: Over the years, individuals may accumulate other risk factors, such as hypertension, high cholesterol, obesity, and diabetes, which further elevate the risk of heart disease.

5. Lifestyle Factors: Aging is often associated with the development of less healthy lifestyle habits, such as poor dietary

choices, sedentary behavior, and smoking, all of which can exacerbate the impact of age on heart disease risk.

Due to these age-related changes, the risk of heart disease rises significantly after the age of 45 for men and after 55 for women. However, it's crucial to note that heart disease can affect individuals of any age, and lifestyle modifications can help mitigate age-related risk.

Gender as a Risk Factor

Gender is another important factor influencing heart disease risk. Men and women can experience heart disease differently, and gender-related factors include:

1. Men: Historically, men have been more likely to develop heart disease at a younger age than women. They tend to have a higher prevalence of risk factors such as high blood pressure and smoking. Heart attacks in men are often characterized by classic symptoms like chest pain.

2. Women: Women are more likely to develop heart disease later in life, typically after menopause. Their risk increases due to hormonal changes and other factors. Women may experience atypical symptoms during a heart attack, such as shortness of breath, fatigue, and nausea, which can lead to delayed diagnosis and treatment.

3. Gender-Specific Conditions: Some heart conditions, like coronary microvascular disease and stress-induced

cardiomyopathy (often called "broken heart syndrome"), are more common in women.

It's crucial to recognize that heart disease is the leading cause of death for both men and women. Gender differences in heart disease risk underscore the importance of tailored prevention and treatment strategies. Regardless of age or gender, adopting a heart-healthy lifestyle, regular medical check-ups, and early intervention for risk factors are essential for maintaining cardiovascular health and reducing the risk of heart disease.

Chapter 3

Assessing Your Heart Health

Assessing your heart health is of paramount importance for several reasons:

1. Prevent Heart Disease: Regular assessments can identify risk factors early, allowing for preventive measures to reduce the chances of heart disease.

2. Early Detection: Monitoring heart health can lead to the early detection of issues like high blood pressure, high cholesterol, or irregular heartbeats, which can be managed more effectively when detected early.

3. Lifestyle Adjustments: Knowing your heart health status can motivate you to make healthier lifestyle choices, such as improving your diet, exercising more, quitting smoking, and reducing stress.

4. Reduce Health Care Costs: Preventing heart problems or managing them at an early stage can reduce long-term healthcare costs associated with heart disease treatments and hospitalizations.

5. Quality of Life: Maintaining good heart health can significantly improve your overall quality of life, ensuring you remain active and enjoy a higher level of well-being.

6. Longevity: A healthy heart contributes to a longer, more fulfilling life, reducing the risk of premature death from heart-related issues.

7. Peace of Mind: Regular check-ups and assessments offer peace of mind, knowing that you're taking proactive steps to safeguard your heart.

8. Family Health: By assessing your heart health, you set a positive example for your family and encourage them to prioritize their heart health as well.

9. Customized Care: Assessments provide a basis for personalized medical advice and treatment plans tailored to your specific needs.

In summary, assessing your heart health is essential for both prevention and early intervention, ultimately promoting a longer, healthier, and more fulfilling life.

Regular Checkups and Screenings

Regular check-ups and screenings play a crucial role in assessing heart health by providing early detection and prevention of cardiovascular issues. Here's how:

1. Early Detection: Routine check-ups, including blood pressure, cholesterol, and blood sugar measurements, can identify risk factors for heart disease. Early identification allows for early intervention

2. Risk Assessment: Healthcare professionals can assess your overall heart health based on factors like family history, lifestyle, and medical history, helping to determine your risk of heart disease.

3. Prevention: Regular check-ups enable doctors to provide guidance on heart-healthy lifestyle changes, such as diet and exercise, reducing the risk of heart disease.

4. Screenings: Tests like electrocardiograms (ECG or EKG), stress tests, and echocardiograms can detect heart abnormalities, like arrhythmias or structural issues, even before symptoms arise.

5. Monitoring: If you have a known heart condition, regular check-ups help monitor your condition, adjust treatment plans, and prevent complications.

6. Timely Intervention: Screening for heart disease can lead to early intervention, such as medications or surgeries, which can be more effective when issues are detected early.

In summary, regular check-ups and screenings are essential for assessing heart health, identifying risk factors, and preventing heart disease or managing existing conditions. It's crucial to follow your healthcare provider's recommendations for these check-ups to maintain a healthy heart.

Understanding Heart Health Numbers

Understanding your heart health numbers is crucial for maintaining a healthy cardiovascular system. Some key numbers to consider include:

1. Blood Pressure: Measured in millimeters of mercury (mm Hg), it consists of two values - systolic (top number) and diastolic (bottom number). Normal blood pressure is around 120/80 mm Hg. High blood pressure (hypertension) is a risk factor for heart disease.

Normal: Below 120/80 mm Hg
Elevated: 120-129/80 mm Hg
Hypertension Stage 1: 130-139/80-89 mm Hg
Hypertension Stage 2: 140/90 mm Hg or higher

2. Cholesterol Levels: Total cholesterol, LDL (low-density lipoprotein), and HDL (high-density lipoprotein) cholesterol are important. High LDL and low HDL cholesterol levels can increase heart disease risk.

Cholesterol Levels(mg/dL):-
Total cholesterol
Desirable: Below 200
Borderline High: 200-239
High: 240 or above

LDL (Low-Density Lipoprotein) Cholesterol:
Optimal: Below 100
Near Optimal: 100-129
High: 160-189

HDL (High-Density Lipoprotein) Cholesterol:
Higher is better; above 60 is ideal
Triglycerides:
Normal: Below 150

3. Blood Sugar: Fasting blood sugar levels indicate your risk for diabetes. Elevated blood sugar levels are associated with a higher risk of heart disease.

Fasting Blood Sugar (mg/dL):

Normal: Below 100
Prediabetes: 100-125
Diabetes: 126 or higher

4. Body Mass Index (BMI): It helps assess if you're in a healthy weight range. Excess weight can strain the heart and increase cardiovascular risk.

Body Mass Index (BMI):

Normal: 18.5-24.9
Overweight: 25-29.9
Obesity: 30 or higher

5. Waist Circumference: Abdominal obesity, indicated by an increased waist circumference, is linked to heart disease risk.

For men:

Elevated Risk: Waist circumference greater than 40 inches (102 cm)
High Risk: Waist circumference greater than 44 inches (112 cm)
For women:

Elevated Risk: Waist circumference greater than 35 inches (88 cm)
High Risk: Waist circumference greater than 40 inches (102 cm)

6. Physical Activity: Regular exercise helps maintain a healthy heart. Aim for at least 150 minutes of moderate aerobic activity per week.

Monitoring these numbers, making lifestyle changes as needed, and working with your healthcare provider can help you maintain optimal heart health.

Keeping a Heart Health Journal

Keeping a heart health journal can be a valuable tool for monitoring and improving your cardiovascular well-being. Here's how you can start one:

1. Record Key Metrics: Regularly log important numbers such as blood pressure, heart rate, weight, and cholesterol levels. Note the date and time for each entry.

2. Dietary Habits: Document your daily meals and snacks. Include details about portion sizes, ingredients, and any special dietary restrictions or goals.

3. Physical Activity: Track your exercise routines. Note the type of activity, duration, and intensity. This can help you ensure you're meeting recommended exercise guidelines.

4. Medications and Supplements: List all the medications and supplements you take, including dosages and frequency. This is crucial for managing your heart condition and avoiding potential interactions.

5. Symptoms: If you experience any unusual symptoms such as chest pain, shortness of breath, or fatigue, record them. Note when they occur, how long they last, and their severity.

6. Stress Levels: Monitor your stress levels and factors that contribute to stress. Identifying stress triggers can help you manage them more effectively.

7. Sleep Patterns: Record your sleep patterns, including the number of hours you sleep each night and any disturbances. Quality sleep is essential for heart health.

8. Alcohol and Tobacco Use: If applicable, track your alcohol consumption and smoking habits. These habits can and will have a significant impact on your heart health.

9. Emotional Well-being: Note your emotional state each day. High stress, anxiety, or depression can affect heart health, so it's essential to be aware of your mood.

10. Consultations: Document your visits to healthcare professionals, including the date, reason for the visit, and any advice or recommendations you receive.

11. Goals and Progress: Set heart health goals, such as achieving specific cholesterol levels or increasing your exercise duration. Regularly update your journal with your progress toward these goals.

12. Reflection: Take time to reflect on your entries and identify trends or patterns. This can help you and your healthcare team make informed decisions about your heart health.

Remember that your heart health journal is a personal tool, and you can customize it to meet your specific needs and goals. It's also a helpful resource when discussing your heart health with your healthcare provider, as it provides them with valuable insights into your lifestyle and symptoms.

Chapter 4

Nutrition for a Healthy Heart

Nutrition is the cornerstone of a healthy heart, and neglecting it can lead to severe disadvantages. A well-balanced diet rich in fruits, vegetables, whole grains, and lean proteins can significantly reduce the risk of heart diseases. Conversely, poor nutrition comes with a host of drawbacks:

1. Heart Disease Risk: Inadequate nutrition, characterized by excessive consumption of saturated fats, sugars, and salt, can lead to high cholesterol, high blood pressure, and obesity – all primary risk factors for heart diseases.

2. Chronic Inflammation: A diet lacking in antioxidants and anti-inflammatory nutrients can contribute to chronic inflammation, a key driver of atherosclerosis and heart attacks.

3. Weight Gain: Unhealthy eating habits often result in weight gain and obesity, which strain the heart and increase the likelihood of cardiovascular issues.

4. Blood Sugar Problems: Diets high in refined sugars disrupt blood sugar control, raising the risk of type 2 diabetes, another major contributor to heart disease.

5. Nutrient Deficiencies: Insufficient intake of essential vitamins and minerals weakens the body's defenses against oxidative stress and inflammation.

6. Low Energy and Mental Health: Poor nutrition can lead to fatigue, reduced physical activity, and even mental health issues, which can indirectly harm heart health.

In essence, the right nutrition is a powerful shield against heart diseases, while poor dietary choices can pave the way for multiple risk factors. Prioritizing heart-healthy eating is a proactive step toward a longer, healthier life.

Heart-Healthy Diet Principles

A heart-healthy diet is a set of dietary principles and guidelines aimed at reducing the risk of heart diseases and promoting overall cardiovascular well-being. The key principles of a heart-healthy diet include:

1. Balanced Macronutrients: The diet should include a balance of macronutrients, including carbohydrates, proteins, and fats, with an emphasis on choosing healthy sources of each.

2. Variety: Incorporate a variety of foods from different food groups.

3. Moderation: Control portion sizes and avoid overindulgence.

4. Moderate Alcohol: If you consume alcohol, do so in moderation. Excessive alcohol can have detrimental effects on the heart.

5. Hydration: Stay well-hydrated with water and limit consumption of sugary and caffeinated beverages.

6. Meal Planning: Plan balanced meals and snacks to ensure they align with heart-healthy principles.

7. Mindful eating: Be conscious of what and how you eat

8. Consistency: Adopt heart-healthy eating as a long-term lifestyle choice rather than a short-term diet.

A heart-healthy diet helps lower the risk factors associated with heart diseases, such as high blood pressure, high cholesterol, and obesity. It also supports overall well-being and can contribute to a longer, healthier life. It's important to note that individual dietary needs may vary, and consulting with a healthcare provider or registered dietitian for personalized guidance is advisable, especially for those with specific health conditions or dietary restrictions.

Foods to Include

Undoubtedly, a heart-healthy diet should consist of a variety of items that support cardiovascular health. Here are some essential items to incorporate:

1. Fruits and Veggies: These are a good source of fiber, antioxidants, vitamins, and minerals. To receive a variety of nutrients, aim for a colorful mix.

2. Whole Grains: Choose whole grains like whole wheat bread, brown rice, quinoa, and oatmeal. They include a lot of fiber, which lowers cholesterol.

3. Fatty Fish: Omega-3 fatty acids, which can lower the risk of heart disease, are abundant in fish including salmon, mackerel, and trout.

4. Lean Proteins Pick lean sources of protein including skinless poultry, beans, lentils, tofu, and legumes. These contain less saturated fat.

5. Healthy Fats' Include sources of healthful fats such as nuts, seeds, avocados, nuts, and olive oil. The cholesterol levels can be raised by these lipids.

6. Nuts and Seeds: Almonds, walnuts, flaxseeds, and chia seeds are full of nutrients that are good for the heart.

7. Dairy or dairy substitutes: Choose dairy products with minimal or no fat, or dairy substitutes like soy or almond milk.

8. Beans and other legumes: These are fantastic options for heart health because they are high in protein and fiber.

9. Berries: Antioxidants found in berries like blueberries, strawberries, and other berries can help your heart.

10. Dark chocolate: Dark chocolate with a high cocoa content may include heart-healthy antioxidants when consumed in moderation.

11. Herbs and Spice: Use herbs and spices for flavor and potential heart benefits, such as cinnamon, turmeric, and garlic.

12. Green Tea: Antioxidants and other substances found in it may help heart health.

13. Oats: Soluble fiber, which is abundant in oat bran and oatmeal, can decrease cholesterol.

To maintain a healthy heart, keep in mind that a well-rounded, balanced diet, portion control, and general good eating habits are necessary. A licensed dietician or healthcare provider can provide you with individualized nutritional advice based on your unique health needs.

Foods to Avoid

Foods that can raise the risk of heart disease and have a negative influence on cardiovascular health must be avoided or consumed in moderation as part of a healthy heart diet. Here are some items to limit or stay away from:

1. Trans fats: These are synthetic fats that are frequently present in processed and fried foods, some margarines, and baked goods. They have the potential to reduce HDL (the good cholesterol) and raise LDL.

2. Saturated Fats: Consuming a lot of saturated fats, which are present in foods like red meat, whole milk, and some tropical oils like coconut oil, might raise your LDL cholesterol levels.

3. Too much sodium: Oversalination can increase blood pressure, which raises the risk of heart disease. Steer clear of salty and overly processed foods.

4. Added sugars: Desserts, sweets, and beverages with added sugars can contribute to weight gain, obesity and heart disease

5. Processed foods: Bacon, sausages, hot dogs, and deli meats frequently have excessive sodium and bad saturated fat content. Instead, choose sources of lean protein.

6. Refined Carbohydrates: White bread and sugary cereals, both of which are manufactured from refined grains, can elevate blood sugar levels and increase the risk of heart disease.

7. Foods That Are Calorie-Dense But Nutrient-Poor, Like Fast Food: Foods that are calorie-dense but nutrient-poor should be avoided.

8. Excessive alcohol intake: Alcohol abuse can be harmful to the heart and general health, even if moderate alcohol consumption may have some positive effects on the heart.

9. Full-Fat Dairy: Saturated fat is found in high-fat dairy products like whole milk and cheese. Select fat-free or low-fat dairy substitutes.

10. Fried and quick meals: These are often unhealthy fat, salt, and calorie-rich foods, which are bad for the heart.

11. Processed foods and canned soups: The salt content of many processed foods and canned soups is high. When low-sodium alternatives are available, pick them.

12. Synthetic sweeteners: According to some research, artificial sweetener use in excess may be harmful to heart health. It is better to use them in moderation.

13. Snacks with a lot of processing: Snack foods like chips, crackers, and crackers frequently include too much salt and bad fats. Choose a healthier snack, such as nuts or fruit.

By avoiding or limiting these foods and adopting a diet rich in heart-healthy choices, you can significantly reduce the risk of heart disease and promote better cardiovascular well-being.

Meal Planning

When meal planning for cardiovascular health:

1. Prioritize whole foods: Choose fresh fruits, vegetables, lean proteins, and whole grains.

2. Limit saturated fats: Opt for lean cuts of meat, and use healthy fats like olive oil.

3. Reduce salt: Minimize processed foods and use herbs and spices for flavor.

4. Include fatty fish: Incorporate salmon, mackerel, or trout for heart-healthy omega-3s.

5. Fiber-rich foods: Embrace beans, legumes, and whole grains to support heart health.

6. Portion control: Be mindful of serving sizes to manage calorie intake.

7. Plan ahead: Prepare meals and snacks in advance to avoid unhealthy choices.

8. Stay hydrated: Drink plenty of water and limit sugary beverages.

9. Consistency is key: Make heart-healthy eating a long-term habit for lasting benefits.

Remember, consulting with a healthcare provider or dietitian for personalized guidance is valuable on your journey to better cardiovascular health.

Chapter 5

Exercise and Physical Activity

Exercise and physical activity are the pillars of cardiovascular health since they provide a wide range of advantages that are necessary for a robust and resilient circulatory system. They have several benefits that go well beyond merely keeping you in shape; they are like a tonic for your heart and blood vessels.

The biggest benefit of regular exercise is that it keeps you at a healthy weight and eases the stress on your heart. It helps to improve your cholesterol profile by reducing dangerous LDL cholesterol levels and raising healthy HDL levels. Exercise is also an effective way to lower the risk of heart disease, manage blood pressure, and avoid hypertension.
But the benefits don't stop there. Physical activity enhances the efficiency of your heart, enabling it to pump blood more effectively with each beat. It also plays a pivotal role in managing blood sugar levels, reducing the risk of type 2 diabetes, a significant contributor to cardiovascular disease.

Furthermore, exercise contributes to better circulation, promoting the dilation of blood vessels and reducing the formation of blood clots. It even aids in stress reduction, a key factor in heart health, and boosts overall well-being through the release of endorphins.

In essence, exercise and physical activity are like a shield for your cardiovascular system, fortifying it against various risks and ensuring it functions optimally. Incorporating regular exercise into your routine is a fundamental step toward a healthier heart and a longer, more vibrant life.

Benefits of Exercise

Numerous advantages of exercise may be shown for cardiovascular (CVS) health. Some of the main benefits are as follows:

1. Stronger Heart Muscle: Exercise regularly strengthens your heart, allowing it to pump blood more effectively with each heartbeat.

2. Enhanced Blood Flow: Widening blood vessels through exercise reduces blood vessel resistance and improves blood flow. This can reduce the risk of hypertension and lower blood pressure.

3. Improved Cholesterol Levels: Your entire cholesterol profile can be improved by exercise, which can increase HDL (good) cholesterol and decrease LDL (bad) cholesterol.

4. Weight Management: Exercise lowers the risk of obesity, which is a substantial risk factor for heart disease and helps maintain a healthy weight, or assists with weight loss.

5. Enhanced Blood Sugar Control: Regular exercise can increase insulin sensitivity and assist in managing blood sugar levels which in turn reduces the risk of having Type II diabetes

6. Reduction in Inflammation Heart disease is at risk due to chronic inflammation. The body's inflammatory indicators can be decreased by exercise.

7. Stress Reduction: Exercise causes endorphins to be released, which can lower stress and improve mental health. Heart health benefits from less stress.

8. Improved Circulation: Exercise can aid in preventing blood clot formation and arterial plaque accumulation.

9. A balanced body composition: Exercise can help you keep a healthy body composition, which lowers your chance of developing heart disease.

10. Improved Heart Health: Exercise can increase heart rate variability, which is linked to improved heart health.

11. Reduced Risk of Heart Disease: Overall, consistent exercise greatly lowers the chance of developing heart disease and associated illnesses including heart attacks and strokes.

12.Increased cardiorespiratory fitness means your heart and lungs can oxygenate your body more effectively, improving your cardiovascular health overall.

One of the best strategies to maintain and enhance cardiovascular health is to include exercise in your daily routine along with a heart-friendly diet and other healthy lifestyle choices. Before beginning a new workout regimen, it's crucial to speak with a healthcare professional, especially if you have any pre-existing medical concerns.

Types of Physical Activity

Numerous forms of exercise can significantly improve cardiovascular (CV) health. These are some essential types:

1. Aerobic activity: This includes cardiovascular exercises like brisk walking, jogging, cycling, swimming, and dancing as well as exercises that increase breathing and heart rate. Aerobic exercise decreases blood pressure, lowers the risk of heart disease, and helps to enhance heart and lung function.

2. Resistance or strength training exercises, such as weightlifting or bodyweight workouts (such as pushups and squats), aid in the development of lean muscle mass and boost metabolism. This can promote heart health and help with weight management.

3. HIIT: HIIT stands for high-intensity interval training. Short bursts of intensive exercise are interspersed with rest or lower-intensity activity in HIIT. This is an effective way to enhance cardiovascular fitness, burn calories, and reducing risk factors such as high blood pressure and cholesterol

.

4. Flexibility and stretching: Exercises like yoga and pilates improve posture, flexibility, and balance, all of which help to protect against injury when exercising and indirectly boost cardiovascular health.

5. Exercises for stability and balance Tai chi is one of these exercises that helps with balance and coordination. Falling can be avoided with improved balance, which is crucial for older persons with heart issues.

6. Recreational and sporting activities Playing sports like soccer, basketball, or tennis may be a fun way to exercise. Both social

contact and cardiovascular health are facilitated by these activities.

7. Regular Activities Daily chores like gardening, housecleaning, or climbing stairs add to your physical activity and, if done regularly, can improve your cardiovascular health.

8. Low-impact exercises: Activities like swimming or utilizing an elliptical machine offer a cardiovascular workout without placing too much strain on the joints for people who have joint issues or who require lower-impact choices.

9. Circuit training: This entails performing a variety of workouts in succession with little to no break in between. It can aid the heart as well as the muscles.

Keep in mind that the finest form of exercise is the one you can maintain frequently and enjoy. A well-rounded strategy for enhancing cardiovascular health might include a mix of aerobic, strength, and flexibility workouts. Before beginning a new workout regimen, it is essential to speak with a healthcare professional, especially if you have any underlying medical ailments or worries.

Creating a Fitness Plan

A proactive move toward enhancing your heart health is developing a workout program for cardiovascular (CVS) health. Here is a step-by-step manual to assist you in creating a successful plan:

1. Create Specific Goals: Specify your exercise objectives in relation to cardiovascular health. You could want to decrease your

blood pressure, lessen your cholesterol, or enhance your aerobic endurance, for instance.

2. Ask a Healthcare Professional: Consult with a healthcare professional or doctor before beginning any new fitness program to make sure it is safe and suitable for your health state, especially if you have any underlying illnesses or concerns.

3. Select cardiovascular workouts: Put some aerobic exercises in your strategy. There are other options, including running, brisk walking, cycling, swimming, dancing, and utilizing cardio equipment like ellipticals or treadmills. Aim for at least 150 minutes of moderate-intensity aerobic exercises per week, or 75 minutes of vigorous-intensity exercise

4. Strength Training: At least two days a week should be dedicated to strength training activities. Weightlifting, bodyweight exercises (such as pushups and squats), and resistance band workouts are some examples of these activities. Strength exercise supports overall heart health by promoting muscular growth, metabolism, and metabolism.

5. Flexibility and equilibrium: Exercises for flexibility and balance should also be part of your regimen. Exercises like yoga, pilates, and stretching enhance posture, flexibility, and balance.

6. Create a weekly schedule for your workouts, including the kind of activity, how long it will last, and how hard it will be. Long-term success depends on being consistent.

7. Warm-up and cool-down exercises Always begin your workouts with a warm-up to get your body ready, and finish with a cool-down to gradually bring your heart rate down and avoid damage.

8. Progression Overload: Increase the length and intensity of your workouts gradually as your fitness level rises. Your cardiovascular system is kept challenged by this gradual overload.

9. Monitor Progress: Record your workouts and note any gains in your general fitness, strength, and stamina. Monitoring your development can inspire you.

10. Nutrition: Include a heart-healthy diet in your exercise regimen. Fruits, vegetables, whole grains, lean meats, and healthy fats are nutrient-dense diets that enhance cardiovascular health.

11. Hydroponics: Maintain a healthy fluid intake both during and after exercise since cardiovascular health depends on it.

12. Give your body enough time to relax and heal in between workouts. Rest days and enough sleep are essential for good health.

13. Seek Support: To increase motivation and accountability, think about finding a workout partner, signing up for a fitness class, or hiring a personal trainer.

15. Regular Check-Ups: To monitor your progress and modify your exercise regimen as necessary, make routine follow-up appointments with your healthcare professional.

Always start slowly and pay attention to your body since safety should always come first. If you are new to exercising or have special health problems, it is always a good idea to get advice from a fitness professional. Long-term success in enhancing cardiovascular health requires that your exercise program be customized to your unique needs and interests.

Staying Motivated

It can be difficult to maintain motivation throughout a cardiovascular (CVS) exercise regimen, but there are a number of techniques you can use to do so:

1. Establish Specific Goals: Establish clear, attainable objectives for your CVS fitness. Having a specific goal offers you something to strive towards and keeps your attention on the task at hand.

2. Mix It Up: Variety staves from monotony. To keep things fresh, try a variety of cardiovascular workouts. Running, cycling, swimming, and group exercise sessions are all options.

3. Locate a workout partner: Working out with a buddy or member of your family may increase enjoyment, motivation, and accountability.

4. Create a timetable: Make a timetable for your workouts and follow it consistently. Schedule your workouts just like any other critical obligation.

5. Follow Your Progress: Use fitness apps or a workout journal to record your progress. Observing progress may be quite inspiring.

6. Reward Yourself: Create a system of rewards for reaching milestones or doing a predetermined number of exercises. Rewards might be modest, such as treating yourself to a movie night or a favorite healthy snack.

7. Join a class or group: Workouts may be made more pleasurable by group fitness courses or organizations that promote social contact and a sense of community.

8. Visualize Your Success. Think about the advantages of your CVS exercise regimen, such better heart health, more energy, and less stress. Visualization can boost motivation.

9. Be Informed: educate yourself on the benefits of exercise for cardiovascular health. Knowing the advantages might help you stay committed.

10. Use Technology: You can track your progress, create goals, and connect with people who are on the same fitness path with the use of fitness apps, wearable technology, and online groups.

11. Establish Mini-Goals: Divide your long-term objectives into more manageable, shorter milestones. Enjoy each accomplishment along the road.

12. Change Your Environment: Occasionally switch up where you work out. Outdoor exercise in various environments may be rejuvenating.

13. Use uplifting self-talk. Positive affirmations should take the place of negative ones. During challenging workouts, remind yourself of your strength and capacity.

14. Maintain Flexibility: Don't be too harsh on yourself if you skip an exercise or have difficulties. It's acceptable to change your plan since life occurs.

15. Seek Professional Advice: Take into account hiring a personal trainer or fitness coach who can offer knowledgeable advice and help you stay motivated.

Keep in mind that motivation might fluctuate. Make use of dedication and discipline to carry out your program on days when you lack inspiration. Exercise can eventually turn into a habit that you actually look forward to, but consistency is crucial.

Chapter 6

Stress Management and Mental Health

We go further into the clinical effects of stress and mental health on cardiovascular health in this crucial chapter. The emotional and psychological landscapes inside of us have a profound impact on the human heart, which is frequently thought of as an organ that works mechanically. We investigate the effects of long-term stress, anxiety, and depression on the cardiovascular system, which can result in hypertension, inflammatory steatosis, and heart disease. Learn the most recent therapeutic approaches and scientific revelations that highlight the crucial significance of stress management and mental health promotion in the goal of a healthy heart. Join us as we explore the complex relationships between the cardiovascular system and the mind.

The Link Between Stress and Heart Health

Stress and Heart Health: A Connection

Stress is more than simply a mental or emotional burden; it is a constant companion in our life. It has a significant impact on how physically healthy we are, especially how healthy our hearts are. This chapter explores the complex relationship between stress and cardiovascular health.

Stress weaves its impact on every beat of our hearts, from the modest increase in blood pressure during a stressful situation to the persistent stresses that slowly damage the cardiovascular system over time. From the production of stress hormones to the inflammation that creates the conditions for heart disease, we examine the physiological mechanisms behind this association.

However, not all of it is bad. We also demonstrate the effectiveness of stress reduction strategies, mindfulness,and resiliency in reducing the negative effects of stress on the heart. We learn more about how managing stress may be an important tool in protecting our most important organ—the heart—as we make our way through this complex terrain.

Stress-Reduction Techniques

1. Mindfulness Meditation: Focusing on the present moment without passing judgment is a form of mindfulness. Stress levels might drop, and mental clarity can increase.

2. Deep Inhalation Breathe deeply and slowly to trigger your body's relaxation response. Deeply inhale through the nose, hold for a moment, then slowly exhale through the mouth.

3. Progressive Muscle Relaxation: To reduce physical stress, contract and then relax muscle units all throughout the body.

4. Yoga: Yoga blends physical postures with breathing techniques, meditation, and stress reduction.

5. Tai Chi: Deep breathing and gentle, flowing movements are used in this mind-body exercise to encourage balance and relaxation.

6. Exercise Regular : Exercise like running, cycling, or walking, generates endorphins that can elevate mood and lessen stress.

7. Aromatherapy Some smells, such as lavender or chamomile, may be comforting. Use fragrant candles or essential oils.

8. Journalizing You can gain perspective and cope with stress by putting your ideas and feelings in writing.

9. Social Support: Talk to your loved ones about your worries. Making contact with loved ones may be therapeutic.

10. Time Management: To lessen stress due to time constraints, organize your chores, establish priorities, and refrain from overloading your calendar.

11. Limit screen time to:Stress can be exacerbated by prolonged screen time and digital gadget use. Establish limits and take breaks.

12. Nature and Outdoor Activities: Taking a walk in the park or going on a trek might help you unwind and relieve tension.

13. Use guided imagery to picture serene and relaxing scenes to lessen tension and anxiety.

14. Art and music therapy: Stress management techniques include becoming creative or listening to relaxing music.

15. Biofeedback: Use biofeedback devices to track and control bodily functions including heart rate and muscular tension.

It is important to search for what appeals to you personally because different tactics may not work the same for everyone. The management of stress can also be accomplished by combining several methods. The regular application of stress-reduction practices can strengthen resilience and enhance general wellbeing.

Promoting Mental Well-being

Promoting cardiovascular (CVS) health is inextricably linked to promoting mental well-being. Not only are a clear mind and emotional balance aspects of psychological health, but they are also essential elements of cardiac health. Here are some ways that supporting mental health benefits CVS health:

1. Stress management To maintain a healthy heart, stress management is essential. Chronic stress can cause harmful habits, increase Inflammation, and raise blood pressure. Stress is reduced through practices like mindfulness and meditation, which is good for the mind and the heart.

2. Emotional fortitude: You can more effectively handle the stresses of life by developing emotional resilience. The effects of stresses are lessened on the CVS system and heart health is enhanced through resilience.

3. Make Healthy Lifestyle Decisions: Making healthy lifestyle decisions is easier when one is in a happy frame of mind. When your mind is in good shape, you're more likely to resist life choices

that are detrimental to CVS health such as excessive smoking, drinking etc

4. Sleeping Conditions: Restful sleep is supported by good mental health. For cardiovascular health, getting enough rest is essential since it helps the heart mend and keep up its regular functioning.

5. Social Relationships: Solid social connections promote mental health and have been associated with a lower incidence of heart disease. Making connections with friends and family fosters heart-healthy behaviors and offers emotional support.

6. Treatment Adherence: People with greater mental health are more likely to follow advice and prescriptions from doctors, resulting in good management of CVS illnesses.

7. Reduction of Inflammation: Chronic emotional anguish can fuel inflammation, a major heart disease risk factor. Lowering inflammation levels can be achieved through promoting mental health.

8. Psychological aspects: The risk of CVS episodes is enhanced by unfavorable emotions like melancholy and worry. Heart health depends on treating these diseases and preserving excellent mental health.

In conclusion, promoting mental health is essential to living a heart-healthy lifestyle and goes beyond simply providing emotional comfort. A peaceful mind supports a strong and healthy cardiovascular system, which eventually results in a longer and healthier life.

Chapter 7

Smoking Cessation and Substance Abuse

Smoking and substance addiction, including the use of alcohol and other drugs, are closely related to cardiovascular (CVS) health. Abuse of drugs and alcohol increases the chance of developing diseases like hypertension and cardiomyopathy by directly damaging the heart and blood vessels. Furthermore, it frequently results in bad habits including smoking, a poor diet, and sedentary lifestyles, raising the risk of CVS.

On the other hand, quitting smoking and dealing with substance misuse are essential measures in preserving CVS health. While abstinence encourages healthy lifestyles, quitting smoking significantly lowers the chance of developing heart disease. Eliminating drug usage can lower blood pressure and enhance general heart health.

Understanding the connection between drug misuse, smoking, and CVS health in this complex web of behaviors and health emphasizes the significance of resolving these problems for a healthier and more robust cardiovascular system.

Dangers of Smoking

Smoking has a number of negative effects on cardiovascular (CVS) health, including:

Smoking is a significant risk factor for heart disease

1. Increased Risk of Heart Disease. It may result in atherosclerosis, which can constrict the arteries and cause heart attacks, angina, and other cardiovascular issues.

2. High Blood Pressure: Smoking can increase blood pressure, which puts additional strain on the heart and raises the risk of hypertension.

3. Decreased Oxygen Delivery: Smoking hinders the heart's ability to perform at its best by reducing the quantity of oxygen that reaches it.

4. Enhanced Blood Clot Risk: Smoking raises the danger of blood clots developing in the blood arteries, which can result in heart attacks or strokes.

5. Blood Vessel Damage: Smoking weakens blood vessels, reducing their flexibility leaving them more prone to inflammation and blockages

6. Good Cholesterol: Smoking can drop HDL cholesterol, a good kind of cholesterol for the heart.

7. Accelerated Heart Rate: Smoking's nicotine content can make the heart beat more quickly, putting more strain on the organ.

8. Arrhythmia Risk: Smoking can cause irregular heartbeats (arrhythmias), which can throw off the heart's regular rhythm.

9. Lessened Ability to Exercise: Smoking lowers endurance and ability to exercise, making it more difficult to partake in physical activity.

10. Secondhand Smoke: Non-smokers who are exposed to secondhand smoke have a higher chance of developing heart disease.

One of the best methods to enhance cardiovascular health and lower these risks is to stop smoking. Once a person stops smoking, their CVS health can drastically improve, and the advantages are seem relatively quickly

Strategies for Quitting

Although giving up smoking might be difficult, it is possible with the correct methods and encouragement. Here are some suggestions for successful smoking cessation techniques:

1. Pick a Specific Date to Stop Smoking: Mark the date you want to stop smoking on your calendar. Setting a goal date might you in your mental acclimatization to the shift.

2. Identify Triggers: Take note of the circumstances, feelings, or behaviors that set off your smoking habit. Stress, boredom,

interpersonal interactions, or certain environments are typical triggers.

3. Look for Alternatives: Instead of smoking, try something healthy, such sucking on sugar-free gum, munching on fruits or vegetables, or doing deep breathing exercises when a temptation strikes.

4. Nicotine Replacement Therapy (NRT): To progressively lessen your need for nicotine, try utilizing NRT products like nicotine gum, patches, or lozenges.
Consult a health care professional for guidance

5. Prescription drugs: Prescription drugs, including as varenicline (Chantix) and bupropion (Zyban), might help lessen cravings and withdrawal symptoms. With your doctor, go through these alternatives.

6. Behavioral Therapy: To address the psychological components of quitting, join a support group, sign up for a program, or get individual therapy. These programs can offer helpful direction and inspiration.

7. Prevent Smoking Triggers: Modify your surroundings to keep out circumstances that can urge you to light up. Remove any smoking-related materials from your house and dispose of your cigarettes, lighters, and ashtrays.

8. Keep Moving: Regular exercise might help you manage stress and curb your appetite. Find a workout program you like to help you avoid smoking impulses.

9. Seek Support: Tell your loved ones about your effort to quit smoking and urge them to be supportive. The company of loved ones can be a source of emotional support.

10. Remain optimistic: Highlight the advantages of quitting, like as better health, greater financial savings, and a smoke-free lifestyle. Every time you encounter difficulties, remind yourself of these causes.

11. Monitor Your Progress: Write down your smoking triggers, cravings, and victories in a diary. This might assist you in spotting trends and marking accomplishments.

12. Have patience: Recognize that giving up smoking is a process, and that setbacks are common. Don't be too harsh on yourself if you make a mistake; instead, see it as a teaching moment and go forward with your quit attempt.

Never forget that giving up smoking is good for your health and wellbeing. You can stop smoking if you're determined and use the appropriate techniques, however it could take some time and effort. Don't be afraid to get expert assistance from a counselor or healthcare practitioner who specializes in quitting smoking if you find it difficult.

Substance Abuse and Heart Health

Abuse of substances, such as abusing alcohol and narcotics, can have detrimental consequences on the heart. Substance misuse can have the following effects on the cardiovascular system:

1. Rapidly rising heart rate and blood pressure are common side effects of several medications, including stimulants like cocaine and amphetamines. The risk of a heart attack or stroke may rise due to this pressure on the heart.

2. Unusual Heartbeats (Arrhythmias): Some chemicals can alter the heart's normal rhythm, which can result in unnatural heartbeats. This poses a risk to life, particularly for people who already have cardiac problems.

3. Cardiomyopathy: Long-term alcohol misuse can cause alcoholic cardiomyopathy, a disease in which the heart muscle weakens and becomes incapable of efficiently pumping blood. This may cause cardiac disease.

4. Atherosclerosis: Smoking and cocaine addiction in particular can hasten the onset of atherosclerosis, a disorder in which the arteries narrow and stiffen. The risk of heart attacks and strokes is increased by atherosclerosis.

5. Increased Blood Clot chance: Drugs like amphetamines and methamphetamines may raise your chance of developing blood clots, which may result in cardiovascular problems.

6. Weakened Immune System: Substance misuse makes people's immune systems more vulnerable, which increases their risk of contracting infections that might harm their hearts, such endocarditis (an infection of the inside lining of the heart).

7. Nutritional shortages: People who misuse substances frequently have poor eating habits, which results in nutritional shortages. These nutritional deficits can damage the heart and exacerbate cardiovascular issues.

8. Tension on the Heart: Substance misuse can cause tension and worry, which can damage the heart. Heart disease risk and excessive blood pressure are both increased by persistent stress.

9. Poor Medication Adherence: People who struggle with drug misuse may not take their heart-healthy medications as directed, which can harm their cardiovascular health.

10. Lifestyle Factors: Poor lifestyle choices, such as an unhealthy diet and a lack of exercise, which are risk factors for heart disease, frequently coexist with substance misuse.

In order to treat their addiction and its effects on their heart health, those who are battling with drug misuse must seek support and help. Advice on treatment choices, rehabilitation programs, and methods may be obtained from medical experts and addiction specialists to reduce the risks associated with substance abuse on cardiovascular health. Making positive changes, such as quitting substance use and adopting a healthy lifestyle, can significantly improve heart health and overall well-being.

Chapter 8

Medications and Treatments

We've covered a lot of ground in the earlier chapters about the complex functions of the heart and the complexities of typical cardiovascular diseases. You've probably developed a thorough grasp of the heart's function as the source of life and the difficulties it may encounter by this point. As we begin Chapter 8, our attention turns to the crucial weapons in the cardiovascular medicine toolbox: drugs and therapies.

Use this chapter as a guide as you set out to achieve ideal cardiovascular health. Here, we look at the drugs that may calm the turbulent waters of high blood pressure, the treatments that can unclog the clogged arteries of coronary artery disease, and the methods that can control the unpredictable rhythms of atrial fibrillation.

The drugs that help lower blood pressure, lower cholesterol levels, and treat cardiac rhythm abnormalities will be discussed in more detail in the chapters that follow. We'll also dig into the realm of invasive techniques and operations that can treat arrhythmias and restore blood flow to the heart. From the drugstore shelf to the operating room, it's a journey that we'll take together, showing the way to greater cardiovascular health.

Common Heart Medications

1. Aspirin: Aspirin is frequently taken to lower the risk of blood clot development and to fend off heart attacks.

2. Statistics: It is recommended to take drugs like atorvastatin and simvastatin to lower cholesterol levels and lessen the risk of heart disease.

3. Beta-Blockers: Medicines that reduce blood pressure and regulate heart rate include metoprolol and carvedilol.

4. ACE inhibitors: Blood arteries are widened and blood pressure is reduced by drugs like lisinopril and enalapril.

5. Angiotensin II receptor blockers, such as losartan and valsartan, which help decrease blood pressure and lessen heart strain.

6. Diuretics: Drugs like hydrochlorothiazide and furosemide assist the body get rid of extra fluid and salt, which lowers blood volume and pressure.

7. Calcium Channel Blockers: Examples include amlodipine and verapamil, which relax blood arteries and lessen the burden on the heart.

8. Nitroglycerin: It is used to treat angina by relaxing blood arteries and boosting cardiac blood flow.

9. Diagoxin: It helps treat some cardiac disorders including atrial fibrillation and strengthens the pulse.

10. Antiarrhythmics: Drugs that regulate erratic heart rhythms include amiodarone and flecainide.

Please keep in mind that these are only broad categories of pharmaceuticals for the heart, and that particular medications within these categories may have various brand names. Always seek the individualized guidance and medication recommendation of a healthcare expert to treat your illness.

Medical Procedures and Surgery

Depending on the individual problem and its severity, many medical techniques and operations might be used for cardiovascular (CVS) therapy. Following are some typical treatments for cardiovascular illnesses, including procedures and surgeries:

1. Stent placement and angioplasty:
   - Percutaneous Coronary Intervention (PCI): A minimally invasive treatment to use a balloon-tipped catheter to unblock blocked or constricted coronary arteries. To maintain the artery open, a stent (a mesh-like tube) is frequently placed.

2. Coronary Artery Bypass Graft (CABG): This surgical surgery uses blood vessels from other parts of the body to build a bypass around clogged coronary arteries. To increase blood flow to the heart muscle, this is frequently done.

3. Cardiac catheterization: An invasive technique to see within the heart's chambers and blood arteries. It can help diagnose and treat conditions such as coronary artery disease, heart valve problems and congenital heart diseases

4. Surgery to repair or replace damaged heart valves is known as heart valve replacement or repair. It is possible to utilize mechanical or biological prosthetic valves.

5. Pacemaker Implantation: This surgical operation places a pacemaker, a device that helps control the heart's rhythm and treats arrhythmias, under the skin.

6. Placement of an implantable cardioverter defibrillator (ICD): A device that monitors cardiac rhythms and administers electric shocks to restore normal heart rhythms in the event of life-threatening arrhythmias, requires surgery.

7. Heart Transplant: In situations of severe heart failure, this surgical surgery replaces the failing heart with a healthy donor heart.

8. Aneurysm Repair: Surgery to strengthen or replace a bulging or weak segment of an artery that, if it ruptures, might be fatal.

9. Electrophysiology Studies and Ablation: - Methods for locating and treating the aberrant electrical circuits that might lead to cardiac arrhythmias.

10. Ventricular Assist Device (VAD) Implantation: This procedure involves the surgical implantation of a mechanical device that assists patients with severe heart failure in pumping blood while they wait for a heart transplant.

11. Transcatheter Aortic Valve Replacement (TAVR): This minimally invasive treatment replaces the aortic valve in individuals with aortic stenosis and is frequently appropriate for those who would be at high risk for conventional surgery.

12. Carotid Endarterectomy: This procedure involves surgically removing carotid artery plaque accumulation to lower the risk of stroke.

Cardiovascular surgeons and experts perform these operations, which are designed to treat certain heart and vascular diseases. The patient's general health, the severity of their cardiovascular disease, and the projected advantages and disadvantages of the intervention all play a role in the treatment decision. To choose the best course of action for their cardiovascular disease, patients should consult carefully with their medical professionals.

Rehabilitation and Recovery

Restoration and recuperation are basic periods of the medical services venture, especially after medical procedures or operations. These stages intend to assist patients with recapturing their wellbeing, strength, and usefulness. Here is an outline of restoration and recuperation:

1. Postoperative Care: After a surgery, patients are firmly observed in a recuperation region. This incorporates checking crucial signs, overseeing torment, and guaranteeing the patient awakens securely from sedation.

2. Exercise based recuperation (PT): Actual specialists work with patients to reestablish versatility, strength, and capability. PT can be critical after medical procedures including joints, muscles, or the cardiovascular framework. It might incorporate activities, stretches, and manual treatment.

3. Word related Treatment (OT): Word related advisors assist patients with recapturing the capacity to perform day to day exercises, like dressing, cooking, and washing, after medical procedure or injury. They give procedures and versatile hardware depending on the situation.

4. Cardiovascular Rehabilitation: This program is for people recuperating from heart medical procedure or overseeing heart conditions. It consolidates exercise, schooling, and advising to work on cardiovascular wellbeing and way of life.

5. Pneumonic Rehabilitation: Intended for patients with lung conditions, this program centers around further developing lung capability, perseverance, and personal satisfaction through exercise and instruction.

6. Discourse Therapy: Discourse language pathologists help patients with discourse, language, and gulping challenges, which can happen after specific medical procedures or neurological circumstances.

7. Wholesome Support: Dietitians might give direction on nourishment to advance mending and oversee persistent circumstances. This is particularly significant in diabetes the board and postsurgical recuperation.

8. Mental Support: Emotional well-being experts can offer close to home and mental help, especially in instances of ongoing ailment, significant medical procedures, or injury. Directing and treatment can assist patients with adapting to pressure, nervousness, or gloom.

9. Medicine Management: Patients might require prescriptions for torment the board, contamination counteraction, or to oversee

ongoing circumstances. Legitimate prescription administration is fundamental for recuperation.

10. Home Wellbeing Care: Now and again, patients get care and backing at home from medical attendants, advisors, or home wellbeing assistants. This can be helpful for people who can't go to a restoration office.

11. Follow-up Appointments: Standard subsequent meetings with medical care suppliers are critical to screen progress, change therapy plans, and address any difficulties or concerns.

12. Patient Education: Training assumes an imperative part in recuperation. Patients and their families are frequently given data about the condition, treatment choices, way of life changes, and taking care of oneself.

13. Slow Getting back to Ordinary Activities: Recuperation regularly includes a staged way to deal with getting back to work, work out, and other everyday exercises. This is custom-made to the singular's condition and progress.

Restoration and recuperation are profoundly individualized processes. The length and force of these stages can shift altogether contingent upon the patient's age, generally wellbeing, the kind of medical procedure or condition, and the presence of any inconveniences. The objective is to upgrade the patient's physical and profound prosperity, work on personal satisfaction, and guarantee a fruitful change back to ordinary exercises.

Chapter 9

Living with Heart Diseases

It's important to manage heart disease carefully and modify your lifestyle. Following your doctor's advice is crucial, as is taking prescribed medications, maintaining a heart-healthy diet, engaging in regular exercise (with your doctor's clearance), controlling stress, and quitting smoking. Monitoring and checkups on a regular basis are essential for keeping the heart healthy.

Coping with a Diagnosis

Although accepting a diagnosis of heart disease might be difficult, there are actions you can do to properly manage it:

1. Educate Yourself: Get to know your disease, available treatments, and necessary lifestyle adjustments. Knowing more enables you to make wise selections.

2. Obey Medical Advice: Do what your doctor instructs, which includes taking prescribed medicine, showing up for follow-up appointments, and getting the required testing.

3. Change Your Lifestyle: Eat a balanced diet, exercise frequently (as advised by your doctor), give up smoking, and drink in moderation to live a heart-healthy lifestyle.

4. Seek Support: Talk to loved ones, friends, or support groups about your thoughts and worries. You can deal with the emotional effects of the diagnosis with the aid of emotional support.

5. Manage Stress: Use stress-reduction methods like yoga, deep breathing exercises, or meditation to assist manage stress, which can exacerbate cardiac issues.

6. Maintain a Positive Attitude: A positive outlook can enhance your general wellbeing. Work toward a healthy future by concentrating on the things you can influence.

7. Monitor Your Health: Keep an eye out for any changes in your health as well as your symptoms. Your medical staff may find this information to be useful.

8. Rely on Medical Professionals: Establish a solid working relationship with your medical staff. They can offer advice, respond to inquiries, and modify your treatment plan as necessary.

Keep in mind that life with heart disease may be managed with the correct strategy and assistance. To live a full life, it's crucial to put your heart health first and make the required changes.

Support Systems

People need support networks in order to manage different difficulties and keep up their wellbeing. These networks of people, things, and institutions offer social, emotional, and practical support. Here are a few prevalent support system types:

1.Family: Family members are frequently a person's main source of support. They provide people a sense of belonging, caring, and emotional support.

2. Followers: Close friends provide support, empathy, and a means of social engagement, all of which can be crucial for maintaining one's mental and emotional well.

3. Mental health professionals: Psychologists, counselors, and therapists provide people with mental health concerns with specialized assistance as they negotiate difficulties and come up with coping mechanisms.

4. Medical Support: Healthcare professionals like physicians and nurses offer medical attention and direction for situations relating to physical health.

5. Community and Social Groups: Joining clubs, organizations, or support groups in your area can provide you a feeling of belonging, connections with others who share your interests, and emotional support.

6. Online Communities: Online forums and virtual communities may bring people together who have same experiences or interests, providing a platform for communication and support.

7. A welcoming work environment: A supportive workplace with considerate coworkers and managers may be a great resource, especially when facing stress or difficulties at work.

8. Spiritual or religious communities: The religion community can offer psychological and spiritual assistance to persons who hold religious or spiritual convictions.

9. Public services and welfare programs can provide persons in need with cash help, housing aid, and other resources.

10. Supportive Therapies: A variety of treatments, including physical therapy, occupational therapy, and speech therapy, assist people in regaining or enhancing their functional and physical skills.

11. Self-Help Resources: Self-help books, websites, and other resources provide people the skills and knowledge they need to handle their own problems on their own.

Building a solid support network is crucial for preserving one's physical and mental health since it may offer consolation, direction, and help amid life's ups and downs. Depending on a person's needs, other support systems may be more effective.

CHAPTER 10

Corrective measures for managing stroke

Immediate Response:
1. Emergency Call: Dial emergency services immediately upon recognizing stroke symptoms.
2. Time Awareness: Note the time symptoms started; it helps guide treatment decisions.

Hospital Care
3. Hospital Admission: Seek prompt admission to a hospital, preferably with a specialized stroke unit.
4. Thrombolytic Therapy (tPA): Administered intravenously to dissolve blood clots.
5. Endovascular Therapy: Invasive procedures to remove or break down clots using catheters.

Rehabilitation and Recovery:
6. Rehabilitation Programs: Engage in physical, occupational, and speech therapy for recovery.
7. Medication Adherence: Follow prescribed medications to prevent recurrent strokes.
8. Cognitive Rehabilitation: Address cognitive impairments through targeted therapy.

Post-Stroke Management

9. Blood Pressure Control: Manage blood pressure within recommended ranges.
10. Cholesterol-Lowering Medications: Prescribed to reduce cholesterol levels.
11. Diabetes Management: Control blood sugar levels through medication and lifestyle changes.

Lifestyle Modifications:
12. Healthy Diet: Adopt a diet rich in fruits, vegetables, and whole grains.
13. Regular Exercise: Follow a tailored exercise program to improve overall health.
14. Smoking Cessation: Quit smoking to reduce cardiovascular risks.
15. Moderation in Alcohol: Limit alcohol intake to promote cardiovascular health.

Emotional Support

16. Psychological Counseling: Seek counseling for emotional well-being post-stroke.
17. Support Groups: Connect with others who have experienced strokes for shared experiences.

Follow-Up Care

18. Regular Check-ups: Attend follow-up appointments with healthcare professionals.

19. Periodic Imaging: Monitoring through imaging studies to assess vascular health.

These corrective measures aim to address the immediate impact of stroke, promote recovery, and manage risk factors to prevent future incidents. Always consult healthcare professionals for personalized guidance and treatment plans.

CHAPTER 11

Curing coronary artery disease (CAD):

Medical Interventions:
1. Medication Adherence: Follow prescribed medications for CAD management.
2. Antiplatelet Drugs: Aspirin or other antiplatelet medications to prevent blood clots.
3. Cholesterol-Lowering Medications: Statins and other drugs to manage cholesterol levels.
4. Beta-Blockers: Control heart rate and blood pressure.
5. Angiotensin-Converting Enzyme (ACE) Inhibitors/ARBs: Manage blood pressure and improve heart function.

Invasive Procedures:

6. Angioplasty: Opens narrowed arteries using a balloon catheter.
7. Stent Placement: A mesh tube to keep arteries open.
8. Coronary Artery Bypass Grafting (CABG): Surgical procedure for severe CAD.
9. Atherectomy: Removes plaque buildup from arteries.

Lifestyle Modifications

10. Healthy Diet: Adopt a low-fat, low-sodium diet rich in fruits, vegetables, and whole grains.
11. Regular Exercise: Engage in aerobic activities to improve cardiovascular health.

12. Weight Management: Maintain a healthy weight to reduce strain on the heart.
13. Smoking Cessation: Quit smoking to decrease cardiovascular risks.
14. Limit Alcohol Intake: Moderation in alcohol consumption for heart health.

Stress Management

15. Relaxation Techniques: Practice mindfulness, meditation, or deep breathing.
16. Regular Sleep: Ensure sufficient, quality sleep for overall well-being.

Monitoring and Prevention:
17. Blood Pressure Control: Maintain optimal blood pressure levels.
18. Regular Check-ups: Attend scheduled medical appointments for monitoring.
19. Blood Sugar Management: Control diabetes to reduce cardiovascular risks.
20. Regular Cholesterol Checks: Monitor and manage lipid profiles.

Cardiac Rehabilitation:

21. Structured Exercise Programs: Supervised exercise tailored to cardiac needs.
22. Education Programs: Learn about heart-healthy habits and CAD management.

Emotional Support:

23. Counseling or Therapy: Address stress, anxiety, or depression.
24. Support Groups: Connect with others managing CAD for shared experiences.

Dietary Supplements:

25. Omega-3 Fatty Acids: Consider fish oil supplements for heart health.
26. Coenzyme Q10 (CoQ10): Antioxidant that may benefit heart function.

Alternative Therapies:

27. Acupuncture: Some studies suggest potential benefits for CAD patients.
28. Yoga: Promotes relaxation and may have cardiovascular benefits.

Continued Education

29. Stay Informed: Keep updated on CAD management strategies.
30. Risk Factor Awareness: Understand and manage factors contributing to CAD.

Remember, individual cases may vary, and consulting healthcare professionals for personalized advice is crucial for effective CAD management.

CHAPTER 12

MANAGING HEART PALPITATIONS

Understanding Heart Palpitations

Heart palpitations are often described as irregular heartbeats, rapid thumping, or fluttering sensations in the chest. While they can be alarming, they are often benign and may result from stress, anxiety, caffeine intake, or hormonal changes. However, persistent or severe palpitations may require medical attention to rule out underlying cardiovascular issues.

Lifestyle Modifications

1. Stress Management: Chronic stress can contribute to palpitations. Incorporate relaxation techniques, such as deep breathing, meditation, or yoga.
2. Caffeine and Stimulant Reduction: Limit intake of caffeine, nicotine, and other stimulants, as they can trigger palpitations.
3. Adequate Hydration: Dehydration can affect heart function. Ensure you are well-hydrated throughout the day.
4. Healthy Diet: Adopt a balanced diet rich in fruits, vegetables, and whole grains. Avoid excessive intake of processed foods and sugars.

5. Regular Exercise: Engage in regular physical activity to promote overall cardiovascular health.

Medical Interventions

6. Holter Monitor: A wearable device that records heart activity over 24-48 hours, helping identify irregularities.
7. Electrocardiogram (ECG or EKG): Records the heart's electrical activity and can detect irregularities.
8. Blood Tests: Evaluate thyroid function and electrolyte levels, as imbalances can contribute to palpitations.
9. Medication Adjustment: If medications are causing palpitations, consult your healthcare provider for possible adjustments.

Managing Underlying Conditions

10. Thyroid Disorders: Treatment of thyroid conditions can alleviate palpitations.
11. Anxiety and Panic Disorders: Psychological interventions, counseling, or medications may be recommended.
12. Arrhythmias: If an arrhythmia is identified, treatment options may include medications or procedures to correct the rhythm.

Nutritional Considerations

13. Magnesium and Potassium Intake: Adequate levels of these minerals are essential for heart function. Consult a healthcare provider before taking supplements.

14. Taurine: Some studies suggest that taurine supplements may have a positive impact on heart palpitations.

Herbal Remedies

15. Valerian Root: Known for its calming effects, valerian root may help reduce anxiety-related palpitations.
16. Hawthorn: Some traditional medicine practices suggest hawthorn for heart health; however, scientific evidence is limited.

Sleep Hygiene

17. Consistent Sleep Patterns: Ensure a regular sleep schedule with sufficient, quality sleep.

Professional Guidance

18. Consult a Cardiologist: If palpitations persist or are severe, consult a cardiologist for a thorough evaluation.
19. Electrophysiological Study (EPS): Invasive procedure to assess the heart's electrical system and identify abnormalities.

Emergency Situations

20. Seek Immediate Medical Attention: If palpitations are accompanied by severe chest pain, shortness of breath, or fainting, seek emergency medical attention.

Remember, the information provided is for general guidance, and it's crucial to consult with healthcare professionals for a thorough evaluation and personalized advice tailored to your specific situation.

CHAPTER 13

Lifestyle Adjustments

Complementing drugs and therapies for cardiovascular (CV) diseases with lifestyle changes is essential. Here are some significant lifestyle adjustments to think about:

1. Dietary Modifications: Adopt a diet high in fruits, vegetables, whole grains, and lean proteins for a heart-healthy lifestyle.
   - Eat a diet low in salt, added sweets, and saturated and trans fats.
   - Keep an eye on portion amounts to keep a healthy weight.

2. Frequent Exercise: Follow your healthcare provider's advice and partake in frequent physical exercise.
   - Exercise helps control weight, lower stress, and enhance cardiovascular health.

3. Smoking Cessation: If you smoke, stop doing so because it increases your chance of developing heart disease.
   - Look for resources and assistance to help you quit.

4. Alcohol Moderation: Keep alcohol consumption to reasonable levels because excessive use might contribute to heart problems

5. Tension Management: To reduce tension, try stress-reduction exercises like deep breathing, mindfulness, or meditation.

6. Medication Adherence: Follow your healthcare provider's instructions for taking any prescribed drugs exactly. Never miss a dosage.

7. Regular Check-ups: Attend all planned doctor's visits and follow-up exams to keep an eye on your health.

8. Weight Management: Retain a healthy weight or, if required, endeavor to achieve it.
   - Losing weight might ease the strain on the heart.

9. Blood Pressure and Cholesterol Control: By using medication and making lifestyle adjustments, you can keep your blood pressure and cholesterol levels within the prescribed range.

10. Carefully monitor your blood sugar levels if you have diabetes. Uncontrolled diabetes can lead to serious complications.

11. Limiting Stressful Situations: To lessen the overall strain on your heart, try to manage or decrease stresses in your life.

12. Social Support: To assist you deal with the difficulties of managing a CV condition, enlist the aid of family, friends, or support groups.

Before making any lifestyle changes, always speak with your doctor since they may offer tailored advice based on your individual needs and condition. Your cardiovascular health and general wellbeing can be greatly enhanced by combining these lifestyle changes with the drugs and therapies that have been recommended for you.

Cardiac Rehabilitation

Following a heart-related incident or operation, such as a heart attack, coronary artery bypass surgery, or angioplasty, cardiac rehabilitation is a comprehensive program created to aid people in recovering and improving their cardiovascular health.

Typically, this program comprises of three essential parts:

1. Physical Activity: Exercise sessions under supervision and with a purpose are part of cardiac rehabilitation. These workouts assist increase overall endurance while strengthening the heart and cardiovascular system. They take place in a secure, monitored setting and gradually ramp up in difficulty to fit individual capacities.

2. Education: Patients are instructed on heart-healthy lifestyle choices, including diet, stress reduction, quitting smoking, and medication administration. People are better equipped to make health-related decisions with this information, which also lowers their chance of developing future cardiac issues.

3. Psychosocial Support: Counseling and support groups are used to treat emotional and psychological well-being. These services assist people in managing their stress, anxiety, and depression, which enhances their overall quality of life and makes it easier for

them to cope with a cardiac problem, which may be extremely difficult.

Cardiologists, nurses, nutritionists, and exercise physiologists work together as a multidisciplinary healthcare team to oversee cardiac rehabilitation programs. It has been demonstrated that taking part in cardiac rehab lowers the risk of further cardiovascular events, enhances patients' physical and mental wellbeing, and makes it easier for them to resume normal activities.

People who have had heart problems must talk to their doctor about if cardiac rehabilitation is appropriate for them since it can be a crucial part of their healing process.

Chapter 13

Prevention and Healthy Aging

For cardiovascular (CVS) health, prevention and healthy aging are essential. A heart-healthy diet, frequent exercise, and stress management are all essential components of a heart-healthy lifestyle. The likelihood of CVS problems rises with age, making lifestyle decisions increasingly important. Smoking cessation, moderate alcohol use, and blood pressure and cholesterol management are crucial. In order to preserve CVS health, regular checkups, medication compliance, and weight control are essential. Adopting comprehensive healthy aging behaviors, such as maintaining a social life and obtaining enough sleep, also benefits cardiovascular health. A longer, heart-healthy life can be attained by putting an emphasis on prevention and healthy aging.

Aging Gracefully with a Healthy Heart

Aging gracefully with a healthy heart involves maintaining a balanced lifestyle. This includes regular exercise, a heart-healthy diet, managing stress, getting enough sleep, and regular check-ups with your healthcare provider. It's essential to prioritize your heart health to enjoy a high quality of life as you age.

Future Trends in Cardiovascular Health

Advancements in prevention, diagnosis, and treatment are projected to be the main trends in cardiovascular health in the future. These possible tendencies are:

1. Personalized Medicine: Cardiovascular therapies are tailored based on a patient's genetic makeup and lifestyle choices to maximize results.

2. Telemedicine: Increasing the availability and convenience of remote monitoring and virtual consultations for cardiovascular treatment.

3. Using artificial intelligence (AI) to improve diagnosis precision, anticipate individual risk factors, and use data analysis to identify cardiac disease early.

4. Wearable technology: Wearable gadgets are being used to continuously monitor heart health and to deliver data and alarms in real-time.

5. Targeted Therapies: Creating drugs and other treatments that specifically target biological pathways linked to cardiovascular disease in the hopes of minimizing negative effects

6. Lifestyle interventions: Putting a focus on the value of stress reduction, exercise, and nutrition in avoiding heart disease.

Regenerative medicine is the study of repairing organs and damaged cardiac tissue in order to heal diseases like heart failure.

8. Precision Nutrition: Individualized dietary programs designed to improve heart health depending on a person's genetic make-up and current state of health.

9. Public Health Initiatives: Ongoing attempts to enhance public health practices and increase knowledge of risk factors like obesity, smoking, and poor diet.

10. Improved patient data exchange across healthcare professionals, researchers, and institutions to better identify and treat trends in cardiovascular health.

By reducing the burden of heart disease, enhancing the general well-being of people as they age, and improving cardiovascular health outcomes, these trends hope to promote cardiovascular health.

Chapter 14

Resources and Further Reading

Here are some resources and reading materials to further explore cardiovascular health:

1. American Heart Association (AHA)
   - Website: www.heart.org
   - The AHA provides a wealth of information on heart health, including articles, guidelines, and resources for patients and healthcare professionals.

2. National Heart, Lung, and Blood Institute (NHLBI):
   - Website: www.nhlbi.nih.gov
   - NHLBI offers research-based information on heart and cardiovascular diseases, as well as guidelines and educational materials.

3. Centers for Disease Control and Prevention (CDC):
   - Website: www.cdc.gov/ncdod/heartdisease
   - The CDC's Heart Disease and Stroke Prevention program provides data, statistics, and educational resources on heart health.

4. Books:
   - "The End of Heart Disease: The Eat to Live Plan to Prevent and Reverse Heart Disease" by Dr. Joel Fuhrman
   - "Prevent and Reverse Heart Disease" by Dr. Caldwell B. Esselstyn Jr.

- "The South Beach Diet" by Dr. Arthur Agatston (focuses on heart-healthy eating)

5. Scientific Journals:
   - Consider exploring medical journals like "Circulation," "Journal of the American College of Cardiology (JACC)," and "European Heart Journal" for in-depth research articles and studies on cardiovascular health.

6. Podcasts:
   - "The People's Pharmacy" and "The Dr. Oz Podcast" often feature episodes related to heart health and wellness.

7. Health Magazines:
   - Magazines like "Harvard Health Publishing," "WebMD," and "Mayo Clinic Health Letter" regularly cover cardiovascular topics.

8. Online Forums and Support Groups:
   - Websites like Inspire (www.inspire.com) and PatientsLikeMe (www.patientslikeme.com) have communities where individuals share their experiences and advice related to heart conditions.

Remember to consult with healthcare professionals for personalized guidance on cardiovascular health, especially if you have specific concerns or conditions. These resources can help you stay informed and make informed decisions about your heart health.

Heart Health Organizations

There are several organizations dedicated to heart health research, education, and advocacy. Here are some prominent ones:

1. American Heart Association (AHA):
   - Website: www.heart.org
   - AHA is one of the largest and most well-known organizations dedicated to cardiovascular health. They offer a wide range of resources, research, and educational materials.

2. National Heart, Lung, and Blood Institute (NHLBI):
   - Website: www.nhlbi.nih.gov
   - NHLBI is part of the U.S. National Institutes of Health (NIH) and focuses on research and education related to heart, lung, and blood diseases.

3. American College of Cardiology (ACC):
   - Website: www.acc.org
   - ACC is a professional organization for cardiovascular specialists, providing guidelines, research, and educational opportunities.

4. Heart Rhythm Society (HRS):
   - Website: www.hrsonline.org
   - HRS focuses on heart rhythm disorders and arrhythmias, offering resources for both professionals and patients.

5. Mended Hearts:
   - Website: www.mendedhearts.org
   - Mended Hearts is a peer-to-peer support network for heart patients and their families.

6.

6. WomenHeart: The National Coalition for Women with Heart Disease:
   - Website: www.womenheart.org
   - This organization is dedicated to supporting women with heart disease, raising awareness, and advocating for better care.

7. Heart and Stroke Foundation (Canada):
   - Website: www.heartandstroke.ca
   - This Canadian organization works to prevent heart disease and stroke through research and public education.

8. British Heart Foundation (BHF):
   - Website: www.bhf.org.uk
   - BHF is a UK-based charity that funds research and promotes heart health awareness.

9. European Society of Cardiology (ESC):
   - Website: www.escardio.org
   - ESC is a professional organization that focuses on cardiology research, education, and guidelines in Europe.

10. World Heart Federation (WHF):
   - Website: www.world-heart-federation.org
   - WHF is a global organization dedicated to preventing heart disease and promoting cardiovascular health worldwide.

These organizations play critical roles in advancing heart health, from funding research to providing educational resources and supporting patients and healthcare professionals. Depending on your location and interests, you can explore their websites for valuable information and resources.

Recommended Books

Here are some recommended books specifically focused on cardiovascular health:

1. The End of Heart Disease: The Eat to Live Plan to Prevent and Reverse Heart Disease" by Dr. Joel Fuhrman
   - This book offers dietary advice and strategies for preventing and reversing heart disease through plant-based nutrition.

2. Prevent and Reverse Heart Disease" by Dr. Caldwell B. Esselstyn Jr.
   - Dr. Esselstyn presents a plant-based approach to preventing and reversing heart disease, based on his extensive research.

3. The Simple Heart Cure: The 90-Day Program to Stop and Reverse Heart Disease" by Dr. Chauncey Crandall
   - Dr. Crandall outlines a 90-day program that includes lifestyle changes and dietary recommendations to improve heart health.

4. The South Beach Diet" by Dr. Arthur Agatston
   - While primarily a weight loss book, it also provides a heart-healthy eating plan that focuses on good fats and low-glycemic carbohydrates.

5. The Longevity Paradox: How to Die Young at a Ripe Old Age" by Dr. Steven R. Gundry
   - Dr. Gundry discusses the role of diet and gut health in cardiovascular health and overall longevity.

6. The 30-Day Heart Tune-Up: A Breakthrough Medical Plan to Prevent and Reverse Heart Disease" by Dr. Steven Masley
   - Dr. Masley provides a 30-day plan with dietary and lifestyle changes to improve heart health.

7. Heart 411: The Only Guide to Heart Health You'll Ever Need" by Marc Gillinov, M.D., and Steven Nissen, M.D.
   - This book offers comprehensive information on heart health, covering topics from prevention to treatment options.

8. Heart Health for All Ages: A No-Nonsense Guide to Preventing Cardiovascular Disease" by Jonny Bowden, Ph.D., CNS, and Stephen Sinatra, M.D.
   - A guide that covers heart health advice for people of all ages, emphasizing prevention.

9. The Plant-Based Solution: America's Healthy Heart Doc's Plan to Power Your Health" by Dr. Joel Kahn
   - Dr. Kahn discusses the benefits of a plant-based diet for heart health and provides practical advice.

10. The Mayo Clinic Diet" by the Mayo Clinic
   - While not exclusively focused on heart health, it offers a balanced approach to overall wellness, including cardiovascular health.

These books offer a variety of perspectives and approaches to maintaining or improving cardiovascular health through diet, lifestyle changes, and medical insights. Remember to consult with a healthcare professional before making significant changes to your health regimen.

Glossary

A lexicon of several terminology used often in cardiovascular health and medicine is provided below:

1. Cardiovascular System: The body's system for pumping blood and distributing nutrients and oxygen throughout the body. It is comprised of the heart and blood arteries.

2. The muscular organ responsible for pumping blood throughout the circulatory system is the heart.

3. An artery is one of the blood arteries that carries oxygenated blood from the heart to the body's tissues and organs.

4. Vein: Blood veins that return deoxygenated blood from the body's tissues and organs to the heart.

5. Blood pressure: Systolic (when the heart contracts) and diastolic (when the heart is at rest) pressure is frequently used to describe the force of blood against the walls of arteries.

6. Cholesterol a fatty component of the blood that may accumulate in arteries and cause blockages and heart disease.

7. Atherosclerosis: Is a disorder in which cholesterol and fatty deposits build up in the artery walls, narrowing the arteries and limiting blood flow.

8. Heart Attack (Myocardial Infarction): Occurs when the blood supply to a portion of the heart muscle is cut off, typically as a result of a blood clot, resulting in tissue damage or death.

9. A stroke is a disorder in which the blood flow to a portion of the brain is cut off, frequently causing brain cell damage.

10. Cardiovascular Disease: a general word that includes several diseases of the heart and blood vessels, such as heart

11. Hypertension: Elevated blood pressure, which increases the risk of heart disease and stroke.

12. Arrhythmia is the medical term for an irregular heartbeat that can be either excessively rapid (tachycardia) or too slow (bradycardia).

13. Heart Failure: A condition in which the heart cannot adequately pump blood, resulting in signs and symptoms include exhaustion and shortness of breath.

14. Cardiologist: A medical professional with expertise in the identification and management of heart and circulatory problems.

15. An arterial wall weakening or bulging known as an aneurysm can develop into a catastrophic medical disease if it ruptures.

16.The pacemaker is: a little device that is inserted into the chest to manage irregular cardiac rhythms.

17. Stent: a little tube that is placed into a constricted or clogged artery to keep it open and improve blood flow.

18. An echocardiogram is a diagnostic procedure that employs sound waves to provide pictures of the anatomy and operation of the heart.

19. Angina: Chest pain or discomfort brought on by inadequate oxygen-rich blood flow to the heart muscle.

20. Risk factors include things like smoking, being overweight, having diabetes, and having a family history that make it more likely that you'll have cardiovascular disease.

The terminology used most often in relation to cardiovascular health are defined in this glossary.